Luisa Maria Ribeaúx Hernández

Nursing Care Protocol.

Luisa Maria Ribeaúx Hernández

Nursing Care Protocol.

A proposal to evaluate the behavior of preterm labor threat.

ScienciaScripts

Imprint

Cover image: www.ingimage.com

This book is a translation from the original published under ISBN 978-613-9-41113-9.

Publisher:
Sciencia Scripts
is a trademark of
Dodo Books Indian Ocean Ltd. and OmniScriptum S.R.L publishing group

120 High Road, East Finchley, London, N2 9ED, United Kingdom
Str. Armeneasca 28/1, office 1, Chisinau MD-2012, Republic of Moldova, Europe
Printed at: see last page
ISBN: 978-620-8-33559-5

To my mother, for her resolute support in the most difficult moments.

To Professor Dr. Juan Carlos Martínez who guided me in my professional development and contributed with his knowledge to the achievement of satisfactory maternal and infant indicators in our unit.

To my father, for his concern, trust and unconditional support.

To Master Ada Núñez Galán, who has been a guide in my professional development, for her knowledge and unconditional help during the completion of this research.

To Professors Abelardo Toirac Lamarque and José Antonio Casas, for their permanent dedication and devotion to the achievement of excellent indicators for our center.

Luisa María Ribeaux Hernández

To all those people, who in one way or another have made possible the culmination of this research, to all of them, my eternal gratitude.

Luisa María Ribeaux Hernández

SUMMARY

The nurse consists of a fully compensatory system in which she provides and manages care, makes judgments and decisions about patient care. This can be seen in the way this professional acts and in the extensions of his or her functions. A descriptive, prospective and transversal research was carried out with the aim of evaluating the behavior of the threat of preterm delivery and designing a nursing care protocol in the Perinatal Maternal Care service at the "Tamara Bunke Bider" North Maternal Hospital in Santiago de Cuba. The study was carried out in 210 patients who were admitted to the service in this period, with this diagnosis, evaluating the patient's responses after the procedure. The observations in the nursing notes and the independent, dependent and interdependent actions, allowed validating the efficacy of the interventions and the satisfaction of patients and service providers. The procedure will achieve the implementation of a nursing care protocol and the design of instruments for its evaluation in order to achieve the termination of gestation, thus obtaining a live, healthy and uncomplicated newborn.

CONTENTS

INTRODUCTION

The main objective of the community is to promote health and the normal and complete development of the individual. A new perinatological conception of contemporary obstetrics imposes different approaches seeking to improve the quality of life of infants.

Every year, about 13 million babies are born prematurely worldwide. Most of these births occur in developing countries and contribute the largest proportion of the world's annual perinatal morbidity and mortality.[1]

In the records of the Public Health System of the City of Rosario, Argentina, the figure corresponding to preterm births (defined as those occurring before 37 weeks of gestation) has been as high as 78%. Information from industrialized countries reveals similar values, with preterm births contributing 69 to 83% of neonatal deaths. Much of the severe perinatal morbidity is also associated with these births. Respiratory distress syndrome, necrotizing enterocolitis, intraventricular hemorrhage and long-term disabilities such as cerebral palsy, blindness and hearing loss are much more frequent in preterm births. [2, 3]

Prematurity has been a pathology that obstetricians and pediatricians have had to face for years, and little ground has been gained, even in developed countries it is the first cause of perinatal death. Great efforts are being made in terms of research and assistance.[2] Inherent to prematurity is high morbidity and the consequences of a high risk of disability due to neurological and nutritional sequelae, learning disorders or phenomena of poor esteem on the part of the family and society.[3]

Over time, more and more importance has been given to infectious factors in the pathogenesis. Among them we have urinary tract infections, which is the most frequent infectious complication during pregnancy, its incidence fluctuates between 3 and 12%, anatomical and physiological modifications seem to predispose to this high frequency.[3]

The etiopathogenesis remains unknown, but progress has been made in some aspects. Placental problems, infections, immunologic, uterine, maternal, trauma, surgery, fetal anomalies, and idiopathic conditions have been reported. Clinically, they are associated with extreme maternal age, socioeconomic deprivation, history of hypertension, history of prematurity, premature rupture of membranes, fetal growth restriction, toxic habits, drugs, malnutrition, hypertensive maternal diseases, pre-eclampsia, maternal infections, multigestation, assisted fertilization, interventionism, etc.[2] Recently, the role of the fetus in the initiation of labor has been recognized. In a simplistic manner, it is proposed that the fetus, recognizing that its environment has become hostile, precipitates labor.[3]

The incidence of preterm birth remains stable in various regions of the world between 5 and 12%, including some with a tendency to increase. Emphasis exists in Latin American countries, where in general there is a negative impact on the health sector due to current socioeconomic conditions and deficient health policies. The influence of infectious factors is increasingly present. Antibiotics have even been used to stop the threat of premature labor. Approximately 40% of preterm deliveries are due to infectious causes.[4]

On the other hand, preterm birth is associated with significant public health expenditures. In industrialized countries, the majority of low birth weight infants are usually preterm. A study in the United States estimated that additional expenditures on health, education and general care for children aged 15 years or younger with low birth weight amounted to about $6 billion in 2008. Among those born weighing less than 1,500 grams, who constitute about 1% of all births, the cost of medical care for each child during the first year of life averaged $60,000.[5]

Since the triumph of the Revolution, our health organization has begun to carry out an increasing number and quality of activities aimed at the promotion, prevention and protection of the health of mothers and children, which have borne fruit with evident achievements that have been manifested in most indicators, among them the reduction in the rates of Perinatal Mortality I and Infant Mortality.[6]

The work of the Revolution in Cuban Public Health has always given priority to population groups at risk, and thus social and health actions in relation to women and children have been outstanding. The main achievements obtained in the indicators that reflect the state of maternal and child health in Cuba are implicit in most of the social, cultural and economic development actions, within a political will and the non-discrimination of women and children, who enjoy advantages and programs of education, culture and others within the society and that increase integrally the healthy maternal and child state.[7]

In Cuba, one of the objectives of the National Health System is to achieve excellence in the care of mothers and children through promotion, prevention and recovery through the Maternal and Infant

Care program as a health strategy with the aim of reducing the Morbidity and Mortality Indicators in our country.[8, 9]

The health system requires that all those responsible for the care of the population become involved in actions aimed at improving the quality of service in different areas. Quality is as important a value as health; that is why the nursing staff, as a member of the health team, must develop a culture of quality and join the programs with a proactive attitude.[10]

Internationally, there is a trend to create new strategies to guarantee patient safety, as well as to demonstrate the quality of care provided and thus facilitate the creation of evaluation indicators. The safe interventions derived from them have the capacity to produce a positive impact on mortality, morbidity, disability and complications in users, as well as to determine the guarantee of the quality of care.[10]

In this sense, from Florence Nightingale to the present day, nursing has always shown willingness and commitment to patient safety and to continuously improve the care processes it provides. It is precisely her who, in her Nursing Notes, said further on: "All the results of good nursing care can be negatived by a defect, by not knowing how to achieve what is done when one is there, to be done when one is not there" this statement can be recognized as the beginning of the idea of the Nursing Care Plan.[11]

Nursing as a profession is part of the health services, playing a very important role in patient care, getting involved in the social and health reality of our country and coordinating efforts with the rest of the health team in the fulfillment of institutional objectives of the health sector and within the framework of the quality of care and the guidelines that regulate the professional practice.[12]

The nurse consists of a fully compensatory system in which she provides and manages care, makes judgments and decisions about patient care. This can be seen in the way this professional acts and in the extensions of his or her functions. For the nursing staff, given its professional objective, the implementation of the care protocol and the design of the instruments for the purpose of its evaluation in order to achieve the term of gestation, thus obtaining a live, healthy and uncomplicated newborn, is a tool of undoubted value. [13]

Nursing has evolved in a vertiginous and spectacular way as a scientific discipline accepted by nursing professionals themselves and by others who contribute to its work, this profession has two dimensions: science and application of scientific discoveries of care systems, or what is the same, nursing practice and its technical scientific development, this has made it possible to obtain higher levels of competence and performance that address health problems and the satisfaction of human needs. [14]

We have been able to scientifically employ methods and research that have turned nursing in our times into a profession of high scientific level that our staff is able by itself to identify problems, categorize positive and negative data, and from there, establish priorities, make nursing diagnoses, outline objectives and expectations execute independent actions, assessing the patient's response to call these characteristics made, Nursing Care Process (hereinafter PAE), as a scientific guiding method of professional activity.[15]

The nursing profession has been adapting to meet the changing needs and expectations of the different health care services at the three levels of care. This can be seen in the expansion of the functions of this professional. The development of preventive medicine in gynecobstetric care, together with substantial technical and organizational changes to improve the quality of care for the mother-child binomial, have made it necessary to seek dynamic ways to favor the performance of the health team, among which is the early detection of risk factors in pregnant women with threatened preterm labor, both in those admitted to the hospital or home and those who have not required this essential medical indication.[12]

In our unit the incidence of preterm deliveries from 2015 to 2020 has behaved as follows:

- The Hospital Materno Norte "Tamara Bunke Bider", is a hospital center where approximately 75% of low birth weight newborns are attended with excellent results in Infant Mortality (1.2 per 1000 live births). [16]
- In the year 2020 the prematurity rate was 8.1% and low birth weight newborns a total of 252, therefore, the implementation of a nursing care protocol for pregnant women with threatened preterm delivery is an indispensable premise to achieve an efficient professional performance in the Maternal Perinatal Care service (hereinafter CMP). Hence the motivation for conducting this research.

PROBLEM STATEMENT

The public health system aspires to train competent professionals in the performance of their functions, capable of successfully facing all the demands in the current Cuban context, the threat of pre-term delivery constitutes a problem in our province, the satisfactory evolution of these pregnant women is closely related to the nursing care that is carried out and it should be achieved that the pregnancy is prolonged to term obtaining a healthy newborn, with good weight and without complications. Thus, the implementation of a Nursing Care Protocol is a current problem in the training of professionals working in the Perinatal Maternal Care Service.

HYPOTHESIS

The implementation of a nursing care protocol for pregnant women with threatened preterm labor in the Perinatal Maternal Care service will allow strategies to be drawn up to provide a better service that satisfies the worker in his performance and the patient with the care received.

GENERAL OBJECTIVE

To evaluate the behavior of the threat of pre-term delivery in the Maternal Perinatal Care service at the "Tamara Bunke Bider" North Maternal Hospital of Santiago de Cuba, during the year 2020.

SPECIFIC OBJECTIVES

To design a nursing care protocol for pregnant women diagnosed with threatened preterm labor.

THEORETICAL FRAMEWORK

1. At what point in pregnancy are most premature babies born?

Premature birth is a serious health problem. Premature babies are at increased risk for health complications at birth, such as respiratory problems, and even death. In most cases, these babies require special care in a neonatal intensive care unit, with specialized medical staff and equipment capable of treating the different problems they are exposed to.[17]

Premature infants also have a higher risk of permanent disabilities, such as mental retardation, learning and behavioral problems, cerebral palsy, lung problems, and vision and hearing loss. Recent studies suggest that premature infants may have an increased risk of developing symptoms associated with autism (social, behavioral and speech problems). [9,17]

Studies also suggest that very premature babies may have an increased risk of certain health problems in adulthood, such as diabetes, high blood pressure and heart disease. More than 70 percent of premature babies are born between 34 and 36 weeks gestation. These are referred to as near-term preterm births. These babies account for most of the increase in the rate of preterm births in the United States. A 2008 study found that cesarean sections account for virtually all of the increase in singleton preterm births in the United States and that this group had the largest increase in cesarean deliveries. [5,17]

About 12 percent of premature babies are born between 32 and 33 weeks gestation, about 10 percent between 28 and 31 weeks and about six percent before 28 weeks gestation. [2,17] All premature babies are at risk for health problems, but the more premature they are, the higher the risk of serious complications. [17]

Babies born before 32 weeks gestation are usually very small and their organs are less developed than those of babies born later. Fortunately, advances in obstetrics and neonatology, the branch of pediatrics that cares for newborns, have improved the chances of survival for even the smallest babies.

1.1. What are the causes of premature births?

Most preterm births are due to spontaneous preterm labor or as a result of premature rupture of the membranes, when the sac inside the uterus containing the baby breaks prematurely. Premature labor is the name given to labor that begins before 37 weeks of gestation. The causes of preterm labor or premature rupture of the membranes are not known for certain, but the latest research suggests that in many cases they are due to the body's natural response to certain infections, such as those affecting the amniotic fluid and fetal membranes.

However, in about half of preterm births, physicians are unable to determine the reason for the woman's preterm labor.[18] Approximately 25% of preterm births occur when the physician induces labor before term or when a cesarean delivery is performed due to complications in the pregnancy or health problems of the mother or fetus.

In many of these cases, preterm birth is probably the safest option for mother and baby. What concerns the March of Dimes, however, is that some preterm deliveries take place without adequate medical justification or are performed at the mother's request. In some cases, this can lead to a near-term preterm birth with potential risks to the baby. Women are advised to wait at least 39 weeks to schedule an induced labor or cesarean section, unless there are medical problems that require an earlier delivery.[19]

1.2. Which women have a higher risk of having a preterm birth?

Any woman can have a preterm birth, but there are some women who are at higher risk. Researchers have identified some risk factors but doctors have not yet been able to determine which women are most at risk.[20]

- There are three groups of women with an increased risk of preterm delivery:
  - ✓ Women who have already given birth prematurely
  - ✓ Women expecting twins, triplets or more babies
  - ✓ Women with certain abnormalities of the uterus or cervix
- Certain lifestyle factors can put a woman at greater risk for preterm labor, such as:
  - ✓ Lack of prenatal care or starting prenatal care too late
  - ✓ Smoking
  - ✓ Drinking alcohol
  - ✓ Illicit drug use
  - ✓ Exposure to the drug diethylstilbestrol (DES)
  - ✓ Domestic violence (including physical, sexual and emotional abuse)
  - ✓ Lack of social support
  - ✓ Excessive stress levels
  - ✓ Working long hours while standing for too long at a time
  - ✓ Exposure to certain environmental contaminants
- Certain medical conditions during pregnancy can also increase a woman's chance of having a premature delivery, such as:

- ✓ Infections (including urinary tract, vaginal, sexually transmitted, and other infections)
- ✓ High blood pressure and preeclampsia
- ✓ Diabetes
- ✓ Coagulation disorders (thrombophilia)
- ✓ Underweight before pregnancy
- ✓ Obesity
- ✓ Short periods between pregnancies (one study found that waiting less than 18 months between a birth and the start of the next pregnancy increases the risk of preterm delivery, although the greatest risk occurs when less than six months elapse.[20] Women are advised to consult their physician to determine how long it is best to wait in each case).
- ✓ Being pregnant with only one baby after in vitro fertilization
- ✓ Congenital defects in the baby
- ✓ Vaginal bleeding.

▪ There are some demographic factors that also increase the risk of preterm delivery:

- ✓ Non-Hispanic black mother
- ✓ Mother is under 17 years old or over 35 years old
- ✓ Low socioeconomic level.

Even if a woman has one or more of these risk factors, it does not mean that she will deliver prematurely. However, all women are advised to learn the signs of preterm labor and what to do in each case.

1.4. What medical complications are common in premature infants?

- There are a number of complications that are more common in premature infants than in full-term infants:

Respiratory distress syndrome (hereafter RDS): About 23,000 babies a year, most of them born before 34 weeks gestation, have this breathing problem. Babies with RDS lack a protein called surfactant that prevents the tiny air sacs in the lungs from collapsing. Treatment with surfactant helps babies breathe more easily. Since it was introduced in 1990, deaths from RDS have decreased by about half. [20, 21]

Your doctor may suspect that your baby has RDS when he or she notices that your baby is straining to breathe. Often, the diagnosis can be confirmed by an x-ray of the lungs and blood tests. In addition to surfactant treatment, infants with RDS may need extra oxygen and mechanical ventilation to keep the lungs dilated.

They may need to use a breathing machine or receive a treatment known as continuous positive airway pressure (hereafter CPAP), a method of delivering pressurized air to the baby's lungs through small tubes placed in the baby's nose, or through a tube inserted into the baby's windpipe (trachea). CPAP helps the baby breathe, but does not breathe for the baby. Sicker babies may need the help of a breathing machine to breathe for them while their lungs mature. [21]

- **Apnea**.

Sometimes premature infants stop breathing for 20 seconds or more. This interruption in breathing is called apnea and may be accompanied by a reduction in heart rate. Premature infants are under constant observation for any apnea. If the baby stops breathing, the nursing staff will stimulate the baby by patting or touching the soles of the feet.[21]

- Intraventricular hemorrhage (IVH).

Brain hemorrhages are common in some premature infants, particularly those born before 32 weeks gestation. These hemorrhages usually occur during the first three days of life and can usually be diagnosed by ultrasound. Almost all brain hemorrhages are mild and resolve on their own, causing few or no permanent consequences.

More severe hemorrhages can affect the substance of the brain or cause the brain's ventricles (cavities in the brain that are filled with fluid) to dilate rapidly and increase pressure on the brain, which can lead to brain damage (such as cerebral palsy or learning and behavioral problems). When fluid remains in the ventricles, neurosurgeons often insert a tube into the brain to drain the fluid and reduce the risk of brain damage.

- Patent ductus arteriosus (hereinafter PDA).

Patent ductus arteriosus is a heart problem commonly seen in premature babies. Before birth, a large artery called the ductus arteriosus or ductus arteriosus causes blood to bypass the lungs as the fetus receives the oxygen it needs through the placenta. Normally, the ductus arteriosus closes shortly after birth so that blood can circulate to the lungs and absorb oxygen. [22]

When the ductus arteriosus does not close properly, it can lead to heart failure. PDA can be diagnosed with a special type of ultrasound known as echocardiography or with other imaging tests. Babies with PDA are treated with a medication that helps close the ductus arteriosus, although surgery may be needed if the medication is not effective.

- Necrotizing enterocolitis (hereinafter NEC).

Some premature infants develop this potentially dangerous bowel problem two to three weeks after birth, which can lead to feeding difficulties, abdominal swelling and other complications. NEC can be diagnosed by blood tests and imaging tests, such as X-rays. Affected infants are treated with antibiotics and fed intravenously while their intestine heals. In some cases, surgery is necessary to remove injured sections of the intestine. [22]

- Retinopathy of prematurity (hereafter ROP).

Retinopathy of prematurity is an abnormal growth of blood vessels in the eye that can lead to vision loss and occurs primarily in infants born before 32 weeks gestation. PDR can be diagnosed by ophthalmologic examination several weeks after birth. Most cases are mild and the eyes heal on their own with little or no vision loss. In more severe cases, the ophthalmologist may treat the abnormal vessels with lasers or cryotherapy (freezing) to protect the retina and preserve vision.

- **Jaundice**.

Premature babies are more likely than full-term babies to develop jaundice because their livers are not mature enough to remove a waste product called bilirubin from the blood. Babies with jaundice are characterized by yellowing of the skin and eyes. Jaundice is usually mild and generally not harmful. However, if the bilirubin concentration is very high, it can cause brain damage. [22, 23]

Blood tests can check to see if bilirubin levels are too high. If so, the baby can be treated with special lights (phototherapy) that help the baby's body eliminate bilirubin and thus prevent brain damage.

Occasionally, if bilirubin levels get too high, the baby may need a special type of blood transfusion.

- **Anemia**.

Premature babies are often anemic, which means they do not have enough red blood cells. Normally, the baby stores iron during the last few months of gestation and uses it toward the end of pregnancy and after birth to make red blood cells. Premature babies may not have had enough time to store iron. If the baby is anemic, he or she often develops feeding problems and grows more slowly. Anemia can also aggravate heart or breathing problems. These babies can be treated with dietary iron supplements, medications that increase red blood cell production, or blood transfusions.[23]

- **Chronic lung disease or bronchopulmonary dysplasia (hereafter referred to as BPD).**

Chronic lung disease primarily affects premature infants who require permanent treatment with supplemental oxygen. The risk of this disease is increased in infants who continue to require oxygen 36 weeks after conception (i.e., when the weeks of pregnancy plus weeks after birth exceed 36 weeks).

These babies accumulate fluid in the lungs and suffer scarring and lung lesions that can be seen on x-rays. Affected infants are treated with oxygen and medications that facilitate breathing. In some cases, they require assistance from a ventilator, which is gradually discontinued. Their lungs usually heal within the first two years of life, although many children with BPD develop a chronic asthma-like lung disease.

- **Infections.**

Premature infants have immature immune systems that are unable to efficiently fight off bacteria, viruses and other organisms that can cause infections. Some of the serious infections commonly seen in premature infants include, but are not limited to, pneumonia (lung infection), sepsis (blood infection) and meningitis (infection of the membranes surrounding the brain).

1.5 Prophylaxis

Preterm delivery continues to be the "big problem" for obstetricians and neonatologists, both because of the difficulties related to the physiology, pathology and care of preterm infants and because of the long-term prognosis of these children. A great deal of uncertainty centers on the subsequent development of these children. Child psychiatrists and psychologists, in numerous studies, have reported alarming figures such as 60% of preterm infants with brain damage of greater or lesser intensity, so that more and more attention is focused on the possibilities of preterm birth prophylaxis.[22, 23]

Prophylaxis of preterm delivery is not easy, given the lack of knowledge of many of the factors that are related to it, as well as the causes that trigger delivery. However, prophylaxis of preterm delivery is a necessity, not only because of the high mortality found in preterm infants, but also because of the long-term sequelae found in follow-up studies of preterm infants.

In preterm births (gestations of 258 days or less), perinatal mortality is 33 times higher than that observed in term births. However, in order to reduce the frequency of preterm births, every effort should be made to detect obvious causes in order to prolong the pregnancy until the chances of the child's survival have increased without compromising the mother's well-being, and this, although essentially an obstetric problem, is the responsibility of all those who have responsibility for the preterm child after birth.

Maternal complications during pregnancy have decreased dramatically in recent years. Better prenatal care favors normal growth and development of the child, especially when the mother is healthy or when maternal deficiencies are eliminated, correcting those that can be treated. Prenatal care patterns are constantly evolving and cannot be the same for all pregnant women.

To what extent, then, could adequate prenatal care reduce preterm delivery rates? There has been much discussion on this point; while some give it relative importance, others consider that women identified as high risk demand greater and more careful medical attention if the incidence of preterm delivery is to be reduced.[22, 23]

Bruns and Cooper report a reduction in the incidence of preterm delivery among selected high-risk groups by intensifying prenatal care. Griswold considers that improving prenatal care decreases the rate of preterm delivery by avoiding many complications, including preeclampsia. According to Mc Gregor, treatment of anemia should increase the average weight of the newborn.

Donnelly believes that there is no certain evidence that prenatal care significantly reduces the incidence of preterm delivery, although it improves preterm prognosis; therefore, new methods of evaluating prenatal care need to be constantly developed.

Terris does not find an exact relationship between preterm delivery and prenatal care, referring to the work of Eastman who noted that the differences he found in prenatal care between preterm and term mothers may not be due to prenatal care.

Crosse, in his book "Pre-Term Baby", refers that weight below 2,500 g can be due to an aborted pregnancy, growth retardation or a combination of both factors. Pre-term birth, a condition of multifactorial etiology that occurs between 22 and 36.6 weeks of gestational age, is a worldwide health problem with a frequency of between 4 and 9% and contributes to approximately 75% of perinatal mortality. 23 It has repercussions on maternal morbidity and mortality, as well as on the quality of life of surviving children. All this justifies working in the interest of modifying the causes that lead to it and trying to inhibit preterm labor when it is not contraindicated.

Preconception prophylaxis: The following aspects are of special interest in relation to the prophylaxis of prematurity:[24]

- ✓ Sex education to prevent early pregnancy
- ✓ Decrease, as much as possible, voluntary abortion
- ✓ Fight against smoking
- ✓ Treatment of cervicovaginal infections

Prenatal prophylaxis

- ✓ To identify pregnant women with risk factors for prematurity.
- ✓ A clinical and ultrasonographic study of the cervix will be performed according to the algorithm described below.

The pregnant women were classified according to the prognosis for preterm delivery into four groups, applying an individual follow-up algorithm for each of these women.[25]

Classification of pregnant women according to delivery prognosis:

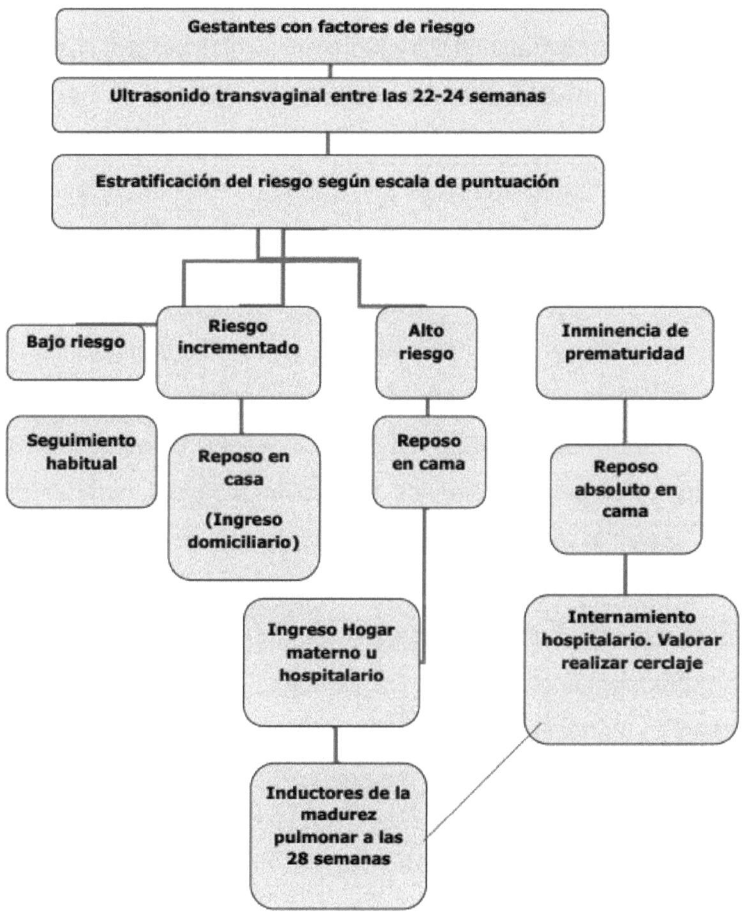

1.6 Assessment of the risk of prematurity due to cervical incompetence:

Cervical incompetence is an obstetric clinical condition, which is attributed with the role of causing late miscarriages and immature and premature deliveries. It consists of the capacity of the uterine internal cervical sphincter to maintain the pregnancy, which progressively yields to the force of gravity and to the hydrostatic pressure of the amniotic sac. Its cause is usually traumatic, provoked by prolonged expulsive deliveries, fetal macrosomia or by abortions preceded by cervical dilatation, it is rarely attributed to a congenital origin. The incidence of cervical incompetence is 2 to 3% of all pregnancies.[26]

The treatment of cervical incompetence, when diagnosed in a timely manner, is simple and consists of a surgical procedure called cervical cerclage, performed between 12 and 14 weeks of gestation.[27] It is necessary to determine the risk factors in a timely manner during prenatal care, in order to reach an accurate diagnosis, using all available means, where the nursing staff's knowledge plays an important role, since they can identify the group to which the pregnant woman belongs according to Dr. Gladys Cruz Laguna's proposal according to cervical characteristics, which will allow them to take actions in order to contribute to the patient's safety.[25-27]

The assessment of the risk of prematurity due to cervical incompetence:

It will be based on the scoring proposed by Dr. C Gladys Cruz Laguna and shown below: [25-27]

A) Cervical characteristics

<table>
<tr><td rowspan="5">Cervical length</td><td>30 mm and over</td><td rowspan="5">It is the measurement of the cervical canal between the internal and external orifices.</td></tr>
<tr><td>29 - 25 mm</td></tr>
<tr><td>24 - 21 mm</td></tr>
<tr><td>20-16 mm</td></tr>
<tr><td>15 mm and less</td></tr>
<tr><td rowspan="3">Permeability of the orifice
cervical internal</td><td>Less than 5mm</td><td rowspan="3">It is the dilatation of the internal cervical orifice, the apex of which is located in the cervical canal.</td></tr>
<tr><td>From 5 to A mm</td></tr>
<tr><td>10 mm and more</td></tr>
<tr><td rowspan="2">Stress test</td><td>Positive</td><td rowspan="2">Cervical foreshortening of 8 mm or more when performing fundic pressure utenna</td></tr>
<tr><td>Negative</td></tr>
<tr><td>Membrane pratrusion</td><td>Yes</td><td>It is the protrusion of the ammotic membranes into the cervical canal.</td></tr>
</table>

b) Score for prematurity prophylaxis:

Cervical characteristics	0	1	*2*	3	4
Longituid cervcal	30 mm and over	29 - 25 mm	24-21 mm	20 - 16 mm	15 mm and less
Permeability	Closed			5*9 mm	10 mm and more
Stress test	Negative				Positive
Membrane pro trusion	Absent				Present

Scoring:

- ✓ Low risk for prematurity that responds to a score of zero to one
- ✓ Increased risk for prematurity two points.
- ✓ High risk of prematurity of three to five points.
- ✓ Imminence of prematurity responds to a score of six or more points.

1.7. Behavior

The following general conduct should be followed:[25-27]

1. **Admission to the Perinatal Maternity Care Ward**

    2. Assess the contractile pattern for 1 hour.

        - ✓ If contractile pattern is normal: Evaluate the pregnant woman and assess whether or not she should remain in this service.
        - ✓ If this is pathological:

1. Proceed accordingly as indicated below.

The possibilities of stopping preterm labor are limited; on the other hand, preterm labor may be a protective mechanism when a fetus is threatened by placental insufficiency or infection. Therefore, trying to stop preterm labor is limited to those cases that could benefit from the use of glucocorticoids.

Pregnant women in whom preterm labor should not be stopped

- ✓ Advanced labor (dilation > 4cm)
- ✓ Chorioamnionitis
- ✓ Maternal decompensated disease
- ✓ Congenital and chromosomal abnormalities
- ✓ Gestation = 34 weeks

Pregnant women with conditions to evaluate for preterm labor detection:

- ✓ Absence of: Infection and/or fever
- ✓ Lack of cervical modifications
- ✓ Pulmonary immaturity
- ✓ Gestational age less than 34 weeks

Behavior according to gestational age and fetal weight:

1. Gestation < 27 weeks:

- ✓ Admission to the Maternal Perinatal Care Ward at 26 weeks and beyond, whenever possible.
- ✓ General nursing measures
- ✓ Sepsis profile
- ✓ Etiological treatment

2. Gestation between 28 and 34 weeks

- ✓ CMP membership
- ✓ General measurements:
  - Rest in left lateral decubitus,
  - Sterile dressing,
  - Nursing observation every 4 hours,
  - Medical evolution each/4hora,
  - Blood Pressure,
  - Respiratory frequency,
  - Uterine Dynamics and Frequency,
  - Cardiaca Fetal every 30 minutes for the duration of the attack tocolytic treatment.
- ✓ Respiratory frequency and osteotendinous reflexes every 30 minutes if Magnesium Sulfate (SO4Mg) is used.
- ✓ Sepsis profile:
  - Hemogram with differential
  - Erythrocyte sedimentation
  - C-reactive protein
  - Vaginal swab with culture
  - Urine cultures
  - Ultrasound:
- ✓ Transabdominal: Biometry, CPF, ILA, PBF.
- ✓ Transvaginal: Look for cervical changes.

Etiological treatment (Treatment of urinary tract infection, vaginal sepsis, anemia, etc.)

3. Gestation = 34 weeks:

- ✓ CMP room admission
- ✓ General measures
  - Resting in left lateral decubitus position
  - Sterile dressing
  - Nursing observation every 4 hours
  - Medical evolution every 4 hours

Sepsis profile

- ✓ Hemogram with differential
- ✓ Erythrocyte sedimentation
- ✓ C-reactive protein
- ✓ Vaginal swab with culture
- ✓ Urine cultures

Ultrasonography: biometry, fetal weight calculation, amniotic fluid index (AFI) and fetal well-being tests (FWT):

Etiological treatment (treatment of urinary and vaginal sepsis, anemia, etc.).

- ✓ Stop preterm labor, she will remain in the CMP room for 48 hours.
- ✓ Subsequently, she will be transferred to the maternity ward.
- ✓ If labor does not stop, it will be allowed to progress spontaneously.
- ✓ Antibiotic therapy: Same scheme as mentioned above.

Knowledge of early diagnosis of threatened preterm labor:

- ✓ Presence of frequent, regular, rhythmic contractions (after 22) before 37 weeks, with frequency between 5 and 8 minutes or less) or exceeding the contractile pattern.
- ✓ Cervical modifications described above.
- ✓ Other warning signs vaginal leakage, decreased presentation, USTV results, among others.

Antimicrobials:

In cases of threatened preterm labor, the macrolide of choice is azithromycin 500 mg every 12 hours for three days or erythromycin 250 mg orally every 6 hours for 7 to 10 days.

Failure of uteroinhibition or its contraindication makes it necessary to face preterm labor. The risks of hypoxia, infection and trauma make it necessary to take extreme care in assisting preterm labor.

METHODOLOGICAL DESIGN OF THE RESEARCH

As general characteristics of the research, it is stated that a descriptive, prospective and transversal study was carried out with the objective of evaluating the behavior of the Threat of Pre-term Childbirth and designing a nursing care protocol in the Perinatal Maternal Care service at the "Tamara Bunke Bider" North Maternal Hospital in Santiago de Cuba, during one year, since this service is the important link in the strategy of sustainability and reduction of the indicators of the Maternal and Infant Program.

Bioethical aspects of research

Ethical principles and patient autonomy were present in the realization of this study. Legal and ethical norms were complied with in order to provide health care with a firm humanistic attitude and legal responsibility.

A form was given to each patient who participated in the study, complying with the principle of respect for dignity, through the right to self-determination and complete information, after explaining the importance of the research, as well as the right to leave the study if desired, elements where informed consent was used as a fair principle, we preserved the patient's privacy, guaranteed by anonymity, (Annex 1).

Universe

It was constituted by the total number of patients attended at the Maternal Perinatal Care service of the hospital, with the diagnosis of threatened preterm delivery during the year 2020, totaling 210 patients:

Inclusion criteria:

- ✓ Acceptance to participate in the study
- ✓ Being admitted to the Maternal Perinatal Care service with a diagnosis of threatened preterm labor.
- ✓ Referred from on-call or other hospital services
- ✓ Gestational age from 27 to 36.6 weeks

Exclusion criteria:

- ✓ Failure to meet the aforementioned inclusion criteria.
- ✓ Patients who were concluded as Transient Oxytocin Discharge.

Exit criteria:

- ✓ Death
- ✓ Transfer to another institution

General aspects of the study:

A form was prepared for the collection of primary data for the proposed objectives (Annex 2). The researcher collected the information provided by the patient's clinical history, evaluating the effectiveness of the treatment through the daily summary note recorded by the nurse.

Biases:

In any study of this type there is the possibility of introducing errors that alter the estimates of the risk associated with the exposure under study. Some of the most frequent errors are mentioned below:

- ✓ **Selection bias:** Occurs when there is an unequal inclusion of cases. In this study such an error is minimized to its minimum expression because it is the same condition since the patients admitted to the Perinatal Maternal Care service with the diagnosis of Threatened Preterm Labor will be evaluated.

For this study, a conventional treatment of obligatory compliance and global accessibility for all patients, not only in the province of Santiago de Cuba but also in the whole country, was performed, therefore, this also reduces the detection bias since each patient is given this treatment. It is possible that the bias of non-respondents may occur, since this research requires the consent or voluntary participation of the patients. There is also the possibility of inclusion-exclusion bias, and to avoid this we created a registry of patients included and not included in the study.

- ✓ **Observer bias:** In a study of this type, knowledge on the part of the researcher may bias primary data collection, especially when the research problem is known.
- ✓ **Error in the classification of the disease:** This error will be minimized through the confirmation of the diagnosis and evolutionary follow-up of the patients with threatened preterm labor through the survey applied by the author to each patient. There is also no possibility of the occurrence of the protopathic seal, since the temporal origin approach is very clear, i.e., factors (represented as a variable) are investigated.

OPERATIONALIZATION OF VARIABLES

Age: According to years of age

- ✓ 19 years old and younger
- ✓ 20-34 years
- ✓ 35 years or more

Parity:

- ✓ Primiparous
- ✓ Multiparous

For the qualitative variable mother's occupation and marital status we will consider the following:

Mother's occupation:

- ✓ Housewife
- ✓ Worker
- ✓ Student

Mother's marital status:

- ✓ Single
- ✓ Married

Gestational age:

- ✓ Between 27 and 34 weeks
- ✓ Between 34.1 and 36.6 weeks

Newborn birth weight:

- ✓ Less than 2500 grams
- ✓ Greater than 2500 grams

Pregnancy-associated diseases

- ✓ Anemias
- ✓ Cervical vaginal infections
- ✓ Urinary tract infections
- ✓ Hypertensive disorders
- ✓ Cervical incompetence.
- ✓ Retroplacental hematoma
- ✓ Choriamnionitis
- ✓ Premature rupture of membranes (RPM)

Obstetric history

- ✓ Early primiparity
- ✓ Previous spontaneous preterm labor
- ✓ Previous induced abortions
- ✓ Previous miscarriages in the second semester
- ✓ Twin pregnancy
- ✓ Undersized
- ✓ Short intergenesis periods
- ✓ Others

Administration of the tocolytic

- ✓ Yes
- ✓ No

Presence of adverse reaction during administration

- ✓ Yes
- ✓ No

Application of the nursing care process: Recorded in the clinical history.

- ✓ Yes
- ✓ No

Nursing Actions: As outlined in the action plan.

- ✓ Independent: These are all those procedures or ways of acting, which the nursing staff executes independently (without medical order), with the purpose of alleviating, improving or eliminating the patient's problem in the shortest possible time.

They can be:

- Psychological support actions
- Guiding actions
- Evaluative actions

- ✓ Dependents: Compliance with medical treatment
- ✓ Interdependent: They allow assisting the patient in the different tests indicated.

Some definitions: [28]

- Live birth: The expulsion or extraction of the product of conception, regardless of the duration of the pregnancy, which after separation from the mother breathes or gives any other sign of life, whether or not the umbilical cord has been cut or the placenta has been detached.
- Term newborn: A newborn born between 37 weeks and less than 42 weeks.
- Pre-term newborn: A newborn born before 37 weeks of gestational age.

- Immature newborn: Live birth weighing less than 1000 grams, usually less than 28 weeks gestational age.
- Low birth weight newborn: A newborn weighing 2500 grams at birth, regardless of gestational age.
- Low birth weight for gestational age: A newborn born with a birth weight below the 10th percentile of the intrauterine weight curve, according to gestational age, regardless of the duration of gestation.
- Intermediate fetal death: Fetal death in which the fetus weighs 500 to 900 grams at birth, equivalent to 20 to 27 weeks of gestational age.
- Late fetal death: Fetal death in which the fetus weighs 1000 grams or more, equivalent to 28 weeks of gestational age.
- Perinatal mortality: Includes fetal deaths of 1000 grams or more of birth weight, and neonates who died before 7 days of life, with 1000 grams or more of birth weight.
- Infant mortality: Any live birth that dies before reaching the first year of life.

NURSING INTERVENTION PROPOSAL, FOR PROTOCOL OF CARE IN THE THREAT OF PRETERM DELIVERY

Nursing could not do an efficient job without its decisions being based on deep scientific knowledge of the basic and social sciences related to patient care.[28] Principles are the fundamental basis on which an action is based, and therefore scientific principles are statements of generally accepted facts or an essential truth that can serve as a guide for action.[29]

The basic principles of care provided by nursing depend on knowledge of natural sciences such as anatomy, physiology, microbiology, biochemistry, biology, etc. and social sciences such as psychology, sociology and others. Among these are: [29]

- Helping the patient to maintain his or her personality
- Helping the patient to integrate into society
- Helping patients regain their health
- Protect the patient from injury or external agents or illnesses

The Nursing Care Process provides a mechanism that allows the nurse to make responsible and valid judgments about patients, from which to assess, diagnose, plan, implement and evaluate nursing care in response to the changing needs of the individual. [30]

It is important to note that in the midst of the pressures and constraints of daily practice, when human life may be in danger, it is quite difficult to observe the facts calmly and make logical judgments.[31]

The scientific method is used in other disciplines to solve problems that arise in the field and as a basis from which to formulate research that expands its foundation. Since nursing also aims to expand its theoretical base so that it provides a good foundation for practice, it is important that this process has a scientific foundation.[32]

The application of the process has two parts.

- It is a method that is part of the nurse's nature, in order to make quick and appropriate decisions and reach conclusions.
- It constitutes a scientific method to solve problems, which is fundamental in any profession.

The Nursing Care Process, as it has developed and improved over time, is currently divided into three stages:

- Valuation
- Intervention
- Evaluation

In collecting the data, priorities should be established taking into account the levels of the hierarchy of needs designed by Kalish.[30-32]

Needs affected:

- ✓ Need for security (protection).
- ✓ Pain avoidance
- ✓ Self-realization (concern)

For the adequate follow-up and evaluation of the cases, the nursing actions described below were carried out. The critical path of the Nursing Care Process (P.A.E.) was followed.[30, 31]

Nursing (P.A.E.).[30, 31]

Stages of the scientific method.	Nursing Actions
EVALUATION	• Collect subjective and objective data. • Identify and describe lower abdominal pain. • State the nursing diagnosis.
INTERVENTION	• Set expectations • Compliance with the medical treatment and formulation of the care plan (dependent, independent, interdependent actions). • Monitor the effectiveness of the procedure. • Re-evaluate treatment with the practitioner when expectations are not met. • Fulfill a new treatment and state new nursing expectations.
EVALUATION	• To reflect the evolution of the patient taking into account the changes producedi: Maintains pain. Decreased pain. Elimination of pain.

In this pathology it would develop as follows:

According to the World Health Organization (Bristol 1972), preterm birth is any birth that occurs before the 37th week of gestation (less than 259 days), starting from the first day of the last menstrual period. The lower limit of preterm birth is the 20th week of gestation; any birth that occurs before this time is considered non-viable. Newborns weighing less than 2500 grams are not included in this definition.[33]

Nursing Assessment

Preterm births occur in 5 to 10% of pregnancies. Preterm birth is a major problem as it is associated with more than 75% of perinatal mortality, in addition to high morbidity and long-term prognosis of these children. Newborns born at less than 32 weeks are the most likely to develop neonatal disorders and account for 75% of neonatal deaths that are not caused by malformations.[33]

Causes.

1. The causes of preterm labor are not known, but there are several circumstances related to these. It has been divided into 4 groups that bring together the main maternal and fetal conditions, these are: [24, 33]

- ✓ Conditions or diseases associated with the mother and/or fetus.
- ✓ Placental implantation abnormalities.
- ✓ Hypertensive disease.
- ✓ Retroplacental hematoma.
- ✓ Cervicovaginal and urinary tract infections.
- ✓ Vaginal bleeding in the first 12 weeks.
- ✓ Anemia
- ✓ Cervical incompetence.
- ✓ Uterine anomalies.
- ✓ Polyhydrams.
- ✓ Cardiopathies.
- ✓ Diabetes mellitus.

- ✓ Premature rupture of ovarian membranes.
- ✓ Nephropathies.
- ✓ Hepatitis.
- ✓ Thyroid gland disease.

2.-Without evident cause, about 50% of the cases are of unknown cause, although factors such as the following can be found:

- ✓ Previous spontaneous preterm labor.
- ✓ Age: it is more frequent in those younger than 20 and older than 35.
- ✓ Poor socioeconomic conditions.
- ✓ Maternal underweight and overweight.
- ✓ Low height (related to maternal nutrition, during childhood).
- ✓ Smoking habits (mainly influences the weight of the newborn)
- ✓ Short (less than 2 years) or long (greater than 6 years) intergeneric periods
- ✓ Previous miscarriages, mainly in the second trimester.
- ✓ Previous induced abortions.
- ✓ Fetal death.

3.-Related to multiple pregnancy: about 10% of multiple pregnancies end in pre-term delivery (before 34 weeks).

Induced or programmed: when the fetal extraction is performed because the life of the mother, the fetus or both are in danger.

Among the most relevant factors are:

- ✓ Previous preterm spontaneous deliveries
- ✓ Early primiparity
- ✓ Undersized

- ✓ Poor socioeconomic conditions
- ✓ Smoking habit
- ✓ Short intergeneric periods
- ✓ Previous miscarriages especially in the second trimester
- ✓ Previous induced abortions

Twin pregnancy is responsible for more than 10% of preterm births. When some of these conditions are identified in a pregnancy, this is classified as High Risk Pregnancy, requiring more intense prenatal care, with the aim of decreasing the chances of preterm delivery and prolonging the pregnancy without compromising maternal and fetal well-being.

Among the measures to be taken by the nursing staff are:

- ✓ Early detection and adequate follow-up.
- ✓ Orientation to a balanced diet from the first trimester.
- ✓ Orienting rest is totally or partially limiting physical activities.
- ✓ Determination of ideal weight.
- ✓ Sexual abstinence.
- ✓ Check compliance with treatment for cervicovaginal infections.
- ✓ In case of cervical incompetence, treatment with cerclage.
- ✓ Health education on the signs and symptoms of labor, threat and warning of preterm labor.
- ✓ Prohibition of smoking.
- ✓ Psychoprophylactic preparation for childbirth.
- ✓ Admission at home or in the mother's home.
- ✓ After 28 weeks, reassess the risk of preterm delivery.
- ✓ Early diagnosis of pre-eclampsia, multiple gestation, bleeding and early cervical changes.

The warning signs of threatened preterm labor should also be kept in mind to make an early diagnosis, these signs are:

- ✓ Alterations of the contractile pattern.
- ✓ Presence of cervical modifications in the absence of contractions.
- ✓ Premature rupture of membranes without uterine dynamics.
- ✓ Cervical changes and premature rupture of membranes in the presence of uterine contractions.

The nursing staff at this stage should:

- ✓ Collection of objective and subjective data.
- ✓ State the Nursing Diagnosis.
- ✓ Set expectations.

Nursing Intervention:

The nursing staff should consider the nursing diagnoses proposed below, according to the needs or problems identified.

Nursing Diagnosis, which should be raised:

- ✓ Lack of knowledge about the treatment of their disease, related to inexperience with this disorder.
- ✓ Anxiety/fear related to the development of possible pregnancy complications.
- ✓ Risk of maternal fetal injury, related to the threat of preterm delivery.
- ✓ Pain related to the effects of uterine contractions

The expectations outlined for these diagnostics would be:

- ✓ Acquire knowledge about her disease and express the patient the necessary measures for the control of her disease.

- ✓ Decrease concern and express the patient more security and confidence.
- ✓ Avoid risk of injury and check for signs and symptoms of complications.
- ✓ Disappear pain referred by the patient.

The nurse should.

- ✓ Perform the formulation of the care plan (compliance with nursing actions, dependent, interdependent and independent).

Nursing actions: dependent, independent and interdependent:

Dependent actions

- ✓ Admission to the CMP room when there are warning signs of preterm labor.
- ✓ Evaluation of the contractile pattern (during 1 hour) by medical protocol.
- ✓ Perform complementary tests (blood count, erythrocyte sedimentation, vaginal exudate with culture and urine culture).
- ✓ Ultrasound
- ✓ Use of tocolytics, to stop anticipated uterine activity in compliance with the principles for their use.
- ✓ Compliance with medical indications.
- ✓ Keep in mind the Golden Rules for compliance with drug therapy.

Independent actions.

The pregnant woman should be oriented towards:

- ✓ Knowledge of the risk factors that predispose to preterm delivery and how to reduce them as much as possible.

- ✓ Provide you with information about the signs and symptoms of threatened preterm labor, so that it can be diagnosed early and complications in both mother and child can be avoided.
- ✓ Once the pregnant woman has been diagnosed with threatened preterm labor, uterine dynamics and fetal focus should be monitored.
- ✓ Vital signs should be measured taking into account that the respiratory rate varies, depending on the characteristics of the patient and the medication being administered.
- ✓ Monitor for vaginal leakage and its characteristics.
- ✓ Monitor for pain, frequency and intensity.
- ✓ Observe the appearance of side effects of medications.
- ✓ Improve the nutritional status of the patient by providing her with a diet with the requirements of: vitamins, carbohydrates and proteins she needs.
- ✓ To guide preparation for the different diagnostic tests and complementary examinations, such as hemogram with differential, ultrasound, vaginal exudate with culture, urine cultures, erythrocyte sedimentation, c-reactive protein, sepsis profile, among others.
- ✓ Provide information to the pregnant woman and her family members about her evolution.
- ✓ Provide health education guidance on :
    - Show the correct technique for dressing manipulation.
    - Place the dressing from the vulva to the anus, making sure that it does not move, to avoid dragging microorganisms from the anus to the vagina.

- Explain the importance of resting in the left lateral decubitus position.
- To show the correct vulvar grooming.
- Use condoms during sexual intercourse during pregnancy.
- Explain the importance of personal hygiene during pregnancy and puerperium.
- Inform sexual partners of the importance of treatment compliance and condom use.

Interdependent actions:

- ✓ Monitoring of the effectiveness of the applied protocol.
- ✓ Ask for feedback on the results with the people involved in the study.
- ✓ Re-evaluate with the practitioner a new treatment or behavior when pain persists.

Evaluation:

The nurse should:

- ✓ Evaluate the effectiveness of the treatment.
- ✓ Assess the patient's response.
- ✓ To give finality to the nursing diagnosis when the method is effective and the needs are met.

In the evaluation of the EAP, the expected outcomes, once nursing care is provided, are that:

- ✓ The patient should be aware of the symptoms of threatened preterm labor and report them in a timely manner.

- ✓ Perform oriented rest, decreasing fear and anxiety, since you know about your evolution and the benefits of rest and treatment, medication and collaborate with medical and nursing care.
- ✓ Have a healthy newborn, at or near term and without complications.
- ✓ General measurements.
- ✓ Perform ECP to all patients with threatened preterm labor.
- ✓ Perform nursing observation every 4 hours.
- ✓ Make evolutionary notes as often as necessary.
- ✓ Maintain nursing care protocol.

NURSING CARE PROTOCOL FOR THREATENED PRETERM LABOR AND DELIVERY

Fecha._______Turno.________Edad gestacional._________Peso.______

	Schedules:												
Parameters													
Fetal heart rate													
Uterine dynamics													
Respiratory frequency													
Osteotendinous reflexes, if using So4 mg													
Volumetric expansion (medication and duration)													
Pulmonary maturation (medication and duration)													
Tocolytic (medication and duration)													
Vaginal leakage													
Diuresis													
Others													
Nurse's signature													

First and Last Names: ________________**Cama:**______________________

Room: ______________**Service physician:** _______________________

Parameters to be evaluated by the Nursing staff

- ✓ Fetal heart rate, to be taken every 30 minutes for the duration of tocolysis treatment.

Normal values between 110 and 150 beats per minute 120 and 160 beats per minute

- ✓ Uterine dynamics, to be taken every 30 minutes, for the duration of the attack tocolytic treatment.

Contractile pattern, to be assessed for one hour

Gestational age (weeks)	26	27	28	29	30	31	32	33	34	35	36
No. of contractions per hour	1	3	5	7	8	8	8	8	9	9	9

- ✓ Respiratory rate, to be taken every 1 hour (while administering Magnesium Sulfate).
- ✓ Observe the osteotendinous reflexes, every 1 hour (during the administration of Magnesium Sulfate).

In the case of Magnesium Sulfate, administer 4 to 6 grams intravenously in 100ml of 0.9% physiological saline solution for 30 minutes and continue with 2 grams until uterine dynamics are controlled. Do not administer the medication for more than 24 hours (according to medical protocol).

Monitoring:

- ✓ Hourly diuresis (less than 30 ml per hour).
- ✓ Presence of osteotendinous reflexes.
- ✓ Respiratory frequency (more than 14 per minute).

The nurse will assess osteotendinous reflexes as follows.

1.- Orbicularis oculi reflex. Superciliary and nasopalpebral:

Percussing the superciliary arcade and the root of the nose with the patient's eyelids closed, produces the contraction of the orbicularis oculi and therefore bilateral palpebral occlusion (even if only one side is percussed), it is recommended to perform it with the eyes closed so that the patient does not see the percussive hammer, avoiding that the contraction is produced as a threat reflex and not by the percussion.

2.- Maseterine reflex:

It can be called mandibular (it intervenes in the masseter and temporalis muscles), the patient remains with the mouth ajar and in that position the hammer is tapped directly on the chin, or the index finger of the left hand is placed transversely under the lower lip, well supported against the mandible, and tapped on it. A tongue depressor may also be inserted into the mouth, resting against the lower dental arch, and percussed upon. The response is elevation of the mandible.

3.-Bicipital reflex:

Keep the patient's forearm in semi-flexion and semi-supination, resting on the patient's forearm supported by the elbow, or resting on the thighs, if the patient is sitting, or on the trunk, if the patient is lying down. The explorer rests the thumb of his free hand on the patient's biceps tendon in the ante ulnar fossa and strikes on the nail of the thumb, or on it, with the thinnest part of the hammer hammer, if it is triangular in shape, the flexion of the forearm over the arm is obtained.

4.-Tricipital and olecranial reflex:

With one hand, take the patient's forearm by the elbow and hold it over her forearm, crossing the thorax, placed at right angles to the arm, and percuss the triceps tendon (taking care not to percuss the olecranon), preferably with the wider side of the hammer. The response is extension of the forearm over the arm (tricipital reflex). Another alternative is for the forearm to hang by the side of the body, supporting the arm, in 90 degree abduction.

5.-Supinator longus or brachioradialis reflex:

The upper limb is placed with the forearm in semiflexion with the arm, so that it rests on the ulnar edge of the forearm on the palm of the explorer's hand, or on the subject's legs. Then the styloid process of the radius, through which the tendon of the supinator longus passes, is percussed. The main response is flexion of the forearm; the accessory response is a slight supination and flexion of the fingers.

6. Ulnar pronator reflex:

With the upper limb in the same position as indicated for the supinator longus reflex, the physician lightly percusses the ulnar styloid process tangentially from top to bottom; the response is pronation. This reflex is almost always weak and only its unilateral abolition is of value, or when it becomes very evident in cases of hyperreflexia.

7.-Reflection of the flexors of the fingers of the hand:

The forearm in semi-flexion and supination with the last phalanges of the fingers in slight flexion (the thumb in extension). It can proceed in two ways: the examiner percusses the patient's flexor tendons in the carpal canal or above; on the other hand, he places his middle and index fingers on the palmar surface of the last phalanges of the last three or four fingers of the patient and percusses them. The response is flexion of the last four fingers, sometimes including flexion of the thumb.

8.-Median pubic reflex:

The patient should be placed in dorsal decubitus with thighs apart and legs slightly flexed. The symphysis pubis is then percussed. The response is twofold: an upper one, which consists of the contraction of the abdominal muscles, and a lower one, which is the approximation of both thighs, by the contraction of the adductors of both limbs.

9.-Patellar or patellar reflex. Quadriceps reflex:

The technique can be.

Patient seated in a chair or on the edge of the bed with the feet pendulous, the patellar tendon is directly percussed. The response is leg extension.

2. Patient in bed, the lower limbs are slightly raised with one hand placed under the popliteal bone, thus achieving a discreet flexion of the leg over the thigh, leaving the knee high. The patellar tendon or quadriceps tendon is produced.

10.-Reflejo Aquileo:

The scan can be performed in three different ways:

a) Seated patient: limbs hanging over the edge of the bed, stretcher or chair; the foot is slightly raised with one hand and the Achilles tendon is percussed with the other, taking care not to percute the calcaneus.

b) Patient on knees, stretcher or chair, feet off the edge: the sole of the foot is brought slightly forward and the Achilles tendon or calcaneal tendon is tapped.

c) Lying patient: the foot of the lower limb to be explored is passively placed on the opposite foot in semi-flexion and abduction, resting on its external malleolus; the sole of the foot is taken with one hand and carried in slight flexion, the tendon is percussed. The answer is the extension of the foot.

Indications of Magnesium Sulfate:

- ✓ Pre eclampsia.
- ✓ Diabetes Mellitus.
- ✓ Hyperthyroidism

Contraindications:

- ✓ Absolute: Myasthenia Gravis
- ✓ Relative: Impaired renal function
    - History of cardiac ischemia
    - Use of calcium antagonists

- ✓ Volumetric expansion, theoretically hydration can reduce uterine contractility by increasing uterine blood flow and by decreasing pituitary secretion of antiduicetic hormone and oxytocin.

- Electrolyte solution: 500ml (120 and 160 milliliters / hour: 40 to 60 drops per minute).

If the dynamic persists, after one hour, treatment with tocolytic should be started.

- ✓ Lung maturation: use
    - Betamethasone, 12mg to be repeated in 24 hours up to 24 mg (total dose).
    - Desamethasone, 5mg intramuscularly or intravenously every 12 hours (4 doses).

Any pregnant woman between 28 and 34 weeks at risk of preterm delivery should be considered as a candidate for a single course of corticosteroids.

Contraindications of glucocorticoids:

- ✓ Viral disease
- ✓ Tuberculosis
- ✓ Fever of unspecified etiology
- ✓ Peptic ulcer
- ✓ Decompensated Diabetes Mellitus
- ✓ Hyperthyroidism

Tocolitics

Nifedipidime (10 mg), administer 30 mg orally or 10 mg every 20 minutes until the 30 mg is administered, if the dynamic is stopped, administer 10 to 20 mg orally every 8 or 8 hours for 72 hours.

Contraindications:

- ✓ Auric-ventricular block
- ✓ Maternal hypotension

If tocolysis is not achieved with the initial dose of Nifedipidimo, administer.

B adrenergics:

Fenoterol (0.5 mg ampoule): Dextrose 5% 500ml with 2 ampoules of fenoterol (2ug/ml). Start with a dose of 1ug/ml, (10 drops / minutes). If after 20 minutes uteroinhibition has not been achieved and the maternal frequency does not exceed 120 beats per minute, increase the dose to 2mcg/ min (20 drops per minute, wait another 20 minutes).

Contraindications.

- ✓ Asymptomatic cardiac pathologies.
- ✓ Cardiac rhythm conduction disorders.
- ✓ Hyperthyroidism.
- ✓ Sicklemia.
- ✓ Diabetes.
- ✓ Choriamnionitis.
- ✓ Pre eclampsia - Eclampsia.
- ✓ Maternal hypotension.

Measure:

- ✓ Respiratory frequency.
- ✓ Pulse.

- Vaginal leakage, provide a sterile vulvar dressing and change it every three hours (as many times as necessary), observing its characteristics (color, odor and quantity).
- Vaginal bleeding
- Mucous plug
- Leucorrhea
- Amniotic fluid leakage

✓ Diuresis, will be measured spontaneously every one hour during the administration of Magnesium Sulfate.

Techniques and procedures

Information gathering:

In order to carry out this research, it was previously explained to the heads of the Perinatal Maternal Care Service, with the approval of the vice-director of nursing, the Scientific Council and the Medical Ethics Commission of the Hospital Materno Norte "Tamara Bunke Bider" of Santiago de Cuba.

An extensive bibliographic review was carried out on the subject, coordinated jointly with the experts in the field at the Provincial Center of Medical Sciences through the computerized MEDLINE and LILACS systems, the INFOMED electronic bibliography and the Internet updated on the subject were reviewed, and we reviewed works on the completion of Obstetrics residency at the library of the Information Center. The documentary review technique was applied, from which the form was prepared, the initial data were collected and the final results were obtained.

We also reviewed statistical data from the Hospital Ginecobstétrico Docente "Tamara Bunke Bider" and various publications on this subject both within and outside the country, including our own.

The literature reviewed will be classified into two types:

- ✓ Indirect verification (books, manuals, standards, review periodicals, monographs).
- ✓ Direct verification (original articles).

The bibliography was delimited according to the Vancouver Convention standards.

Data processing and analysis

Once the primary information was obtained, it was processed in an automated way in the S.P.S.S. 11.5 system, installed in a Pentium IV Celeron microcomputer, with this system the calculation of the different parameters was carried out, the analysis of which was performed through the option of this statistical package. The SPSS version 11.5 statistical package was used for the preparation and presentation of the final report.

Discussion and synthesis

In order to achieve the proposed objectives, the information obtained was expressed in statistical tables, through inductive and deductive analysis of the results, the main aspects of interest were highlighted, which were commented on depending on what was published in the available national and foreign bibliographies, which allowed conclusions to be reached and recommendations to be issued in this regard.

ANALYSIS AND DISCUSSION OF RESULTS

Table № I. Distribution of patients according to age group and parity.

	Age group							
Parity	**19 years old and younger**		**20 - 34 years old**		**35 years or more**		**TOTAL**	
	№	%	№	%	№.	%	№.	%
Primiparous	16	7.61	*66*	31.4	54	25.7	136	65
Multiparous	11	5.2	32	15.2	31	14.7	74	35
Total	27	13	98	47	57	40	210	100

Source: Survey

Although childbirth is considered to be a normal process, various adaptations occur during the course of pregnancy that make it difficult to determine the boundaries between health and disease. The well-being of the mother and unborn child is improved when the maternal state is healthy before conception and is monitored in the early stages and throughout the course of pregnancy.

The age of the patients reveals a higher frequency of low birth weight babies in the period of greatest reproductive capacity. About 515,000 women of childbearing age have low birth weight babies each year, mainly in developing countries. [34]

Our study showed that the greatest number of patients were of reproductive age, between 20 and 34 years of age (98 for 47%), a fact that coincides with other authors. Of the 210 patients attended, 136, or 65%, were primiparous.

Several authors have demonstrated a marked relationship between maternal age and the incidence of preterm delivery; Donnelly found, in a study between 1954 and 1961, a higher incidence of preterm delivery in women under 20 and over 30 years of age, citing that Israel noted that preterm delivery rates increase in very young women, especially those under 17 years of age. The cause that triggers preterm labor in these pregnant women may be related to the fact that they are in their first pregnancy, or to an inadequate development of the uterus, pointing out that, in these pregnant women, preterm labor may be due to a failure of the uterus to change from a spherical to an elliptical shape, which leads to disorders in the feto-placental circulation, and may be more related to age than to physical alterations.[35]

It is not clear why women younger than 20 years have a higher rate of preterm delivery. Perhaps the cause is insufficient uterine development, since the incidence of preterm delivery decreases with increasing age in successive gestations.

Table № II. Distribution of patients according to marital status and occupation.

	Marital status					
	Single		Married		Total	
Occupation	**No.**	%	No.	%	No.	%
Housewife	61	30	42	20	103	50
Worker	24	11	17	8	41	19
Student	34	16	32	15	66	31
Total	119	57	91	43	210	100

Source: Survey

Observations from several studies suggest that low sociocultural level, low parental education and higher incidence of family instability with multiple caregivers are associated factors that are more influential than the specific age of the mother. Changes in the maternal life course (leaving welfare and entering into a stable marriage) significantly influence the development of the newborn.[36]

Low socioeconomic status and low nutritional status represented by low pre-pregnancy weight and insufficient weight gain during gestation are risk factors for both preterm delivery and intrauterine growth retardation.[36]

In our study it was found that the highest percentage of patients were housewives, 103 for 50%, 61 of them were single for 30% and only 42 of them were married, it is noteworthy that of the 210, 119 patients were single, a fact that leads them to present socioeconomic factors that favor low birth weight.

Table № III. Distribution of patients according to gestational age and newborn weight.

Gestational age	Newborn weight < 2500 gr.		>2500gr		Total	
	№	%	№	%	№	%
Between 27-34 weeks	21	13,5	4	2,5	25	16
Between 34.1-36.6 weeks	103	66,5	27	17,4	130	84
Total	124	80	31	20	155	100

Source: Survey

Prematurity continues to be the most frequent cause of neonatal death, and there are predisposing factors for preterm delivery such as: personal history and background, concomitant complications with pregnancy, obstetric complications, genital tract and others.[36] Amniotic infection appears as a factor that worsens the prognosis of preterm delivery.[37] The conditions of inferiority in which the preterm infant finds himself before the environment demand special treatment to ensure his survival, since prematurity is possibly one of the most frequent causes of infant mortality and is directly proportional to the degree of immaturity of the neonate. Mortality is highly dependent on birth weight and weeks of gestation.[37]

According to Aguilar, subnormal weight at the time of conception or during the course of pregnancy, as well as overweight of the pregnant woman prior to pregnancy or exaggerated gain during pregnancy, seems to predispose to the delivery of underweight children, as well as to maternal complications; although the weight of the child at birth, in general, seems to be more closely related to the mother's weight at conception than to the increase in weight during pregnancy, a satisfactory nutritional status at the beginning of pregnancy clearly does not protect against the adverse influence of inadequate weight gain during the subsequent prenatal period.[37]

Table 3 shows that of the 210 patients, only 155 had a delivery before 36.6 weeks of gestation, the rest managed to reach full term, that is, 55 patients for 26%. Only 27 of these patients had a newborn weighing more than 2500 grams, for 17.4%, and 103 of these patients had newborns weighing less than 2500 grams, for 66.5%, both groups between 34.1 and 36.6 weeks of gestation.

The size of the child at birth depends on several factors that affect the maternal and fetal environment.[37] The relationship between low birth weight and perinatal morbidity and mortality has long been known. However, it is only recently that the different implications of birth weight in relation to gestational age have been established. Low birth weight infants are of adequate size for their gestational age, but immature because they are born before the pregnancy reaches term.

It has become evident in recent years in preterm services that the problem of prematurity can be solved quantitatively only within really narrow limits. Therefore, the obstetrician must anticipate and recognize those prenatal conditions that often influence both the onset of preterm labor and the survival and development of the newborns. It should be noted that the most frequent newborn complications found in our study were respiratory distress syndrome due to respiratory distress and hyaline membrane disease due to early-onset and presumptive infection.

Table № IV. Distribution of patients according to tocolytic administration.

Tocolitics	№.	%
Nifedipidimo	208	99
Magnesium Sulfate	7	3.3
Fenoterol	5	2.3
Total	210	100

Source: Survey

A review of the literature suggests that tocolysis with beta-adrenergics is effective in arresting preterm labor for a period of 24 to 48 hours. 24 No studies have demonstrated a significant beneficial effect on prenatal morbidity and mortality, prolongation of pregnancy, or birth weight.

Sustained therapy with these drugs leads to a resistance of the tocolytic effect. The administration of beta-adrenergic drugs should be limited to a period of 24 to 48 hours, with the purpose of administering corticosteroids before 35 weeks of gestation.

Principles to be followed in its use:

- ✓ Tocolytics should not cause serious side effects.
- ✓ Stop labor long enough to use glucocorticoids.

Pharmacological agents used to inhibit contractions act:

- ✓ Affecting intracellular calcium concentration in the myometrium.
- ✓ Promoting the removal of calcium from the cell.
- ✓ Depolarizing calcium (magnesium sulfate).
- ✓ Blocking calcium entry into cells by limiting the availability of free Ca++ to contractile proteins of smooth muscle cells.

- ✓ Inhibiting prostaglandin synthesis.
- ✓ Beta-agonists, which combine with cell membrane receptors and activate adenylyl cyclase. The accumulation of AMP within cells prevents phosphorylation of myosin light chain kinase resulting in the prevention of actin interaction with myosin.

Table 4 shows that of the 210 patients treated with tocolytics with an effectiveness of 96.2%, the most used was Nifedipidime in 208 cases for 99%, followed by Magnesium Sulfate in 7 cases for 3.3%, and then Fenoterol in 5 cases for 2.3%. It should be noted that only in 13 cases there was an adverse reaction to Nifedipidimo for 65%, the main symptoms were headache, facial flushing and arterial hypotension, we only had 1 patient with a reaction to Magnesium Sulfate, which represented 0.5% and there was no reaction with the administration of fenoterol.

Table № V. Distribution of patients according to associated diseases

Associated diseases	**No.**	**%**
Anemia	196	93
Cervical vaginal infections	181	86
Premature rupture of membranes	58	28
Hypertensive disorders	51	24
Urinary tract infections	29	14
Placenta Previa	23	11
Choriamnionitis	4	1,9
Cervical incompetence	3	1,4
Retroplacental hematoma	2	0,9
Others	5	2.4

Source: Survey

Prophylaxis of preterm labor is not easy, given the lack of knowledge of many of the factors that are related to it, as well as the causes that trigger labor. However, prophylaxis of preterm labor is a necessity, not only because of the high mortality found in preterm labor, but also because of the long-term sequelae found in follow-up studies.

Maternal complications during pregnancy have decreased dramatically in recent years. Better prenatal care favors normal growth and development of the child, especially when the mother is healthy or when maternal deficiencies are eliminated, correcting those susceptible to treatment.

In our study we found that out of 210 patients studied, 196 of them presented anemia, for 93%, 86% of them had a vaginal infection installed, and 58 of these patients were associated with premature rupture of the ovular membranes, for 28%. Ratten and Beischer,[38] in Australia, noted that the incidence of births before 37 weeks was higher in pregnant women with hemoglobin less than 9.2 g/L.

According to Dana of the New York Laying-in Hospital, preterm labor is usually manifested by rupture of the membranes before onset, finding a 20.2% incidence of premature rupture of the membranes and preterm labor, and he believes that it is not possible to say for certain whether in such cases the forces involved in labor, such as increased uterine contractility with effacement of the cervix, are at work so that PROM is a consequence of these phenomena or whether it is a primary causative factor.[38]

Gunn, in a review on premature rupture of membranes, finds in the literature a frequency of 9% to 40% associated with preterm delivery.[38] Oliva, in a study of 500 preterm deliveries, in 1969, at the "Eusebio Hernández" Hospital, finds PROM associated with preterm delivery in 21.6%. [39]

Lundy, in his study, points out that preterm delivery figures reach 13% to 16%, which is primarily due to PROM.[38]

Baird found that preterm births occur more frequently among women of low socioeconomic status and that these women are generally shorter in stature, postulating that repeated inadequate nutrition in successive generations may be an influential factor. However, Thompson, reviewing the Aberdeen data, finds that of these low birth weight infants, some had a gestational age greater than 37 weeks, suggesting that both genetic and nutritional factors are related to each other, which is supported by studies conducted in several ethnic studies in their respective countries and in these same ethnic groups in the countries to which they have migrated.[38]

It should also be noted that only 17 had a history of previous spontaneous pre-term deliveries, for 8%, the great majority had toxic habits, 181 for 86%, and also regular socioeconomic conditions, 161, for 77%. Cigarette consumption in pregnant women has been studied in relation to pre-term delivery; its action has been evidently demonstrated in relation to prenatal dystrophy, although it has not been shown to be related to pre-term births, that is, it is only as a consequence of the weight definition that it is related to pre-term delivery.

In recent years, a number of careful investigations have shown that etiological factors preceding pregnancy are of great importance. They may act on their own or intervene in the presence or efficiency of the factors that occur during pregnancy, all of which are related to the socioeconomic status of the pregnant woman. Cosgrove points out that preterm births are more frequent in women with low socioeconomic status, where hygiene, diet and cultural conditions are usually below normal standards.[40]

In recent years, a number of careful investigations have shown that etiological factors preceding pregnancy are of great importance. They can act on their own or intervene in the presence or efficiency of the factors that occur during pregnancy, all of which are related to the socioeconomic status of the pregnant woman.

Cosgrove notes that preterm births are more frequent in women with low socioeconomic status, where hygiene, diet and cultural conditions are often below normal standards.[40]

Efforts to prevent preterm labor are aimed at anticipating or detecting risk factors and treating them as appropriate. Interventions to prevent the onset of labor in women at risk are not effective most of the time. Good dietary counseling and encouragement to reduce and eliminate smoking are appropriate interventions for pregnant women in general, but may be particularly useful for women at risk for preterm labor.

Bed rest is beneficial in preventing it, some researchers suspect that bacterial infection of the lower genital tract contributes to the onset of this problem and therefore infection prevention may be helpful in avoiding it. It is also suggested that avoiding intercourse may be a preventive measure, both to reduce the risk of infection and because prostaglandins in seminal fluid stimulate uterine contractions.[41]

Table № VI. Distribution of patients according to EAP application and evaluation of independent actions.

Application of the	YES		**NO**	
PAE	**№**	%	**№**	%
YES	1	0,5	141	67
NO	209	99.5	69	33
Total	210	100	124	100

Source: Medical history

When analyzing table six regarding the application of the PAE and evaluation of nursing actions, we could see that the Cuban Method of Clinical Record of the Nursing Care Process was not applied to pregnant women with this pathology in the Maternal Perinatal Care services, with the application of its three stages.This represented 0.5% of the cases studied; however, only a plan of independent actions was carried out with the objective of satisfying the patient's affected needs, in the form of guidance, psychological support and evaluation, and this is only achieved with the implementation of the PAE.

The quality of nursing services depends on many factors and is closely linked to the competence and performance of the health team providing care and the results achieved by the latter in improving the health status of the population. Providing safe care responds to a professional mode of action, an essential element in the culture of quality that is stamped on health services. Patient safety implies legal and moral responsibility in practice, competent and safe practice of the profession (without negligence and malpractice), as well as self-determination and self-regulation.[13]

This implies a proper assessment of the people who intend to practice the profession and, to this end, the right candidates must be selected, since an activity, which aims to achieve professional status, cannot be allowed to be considered as a refuge for those who do not have the vocation, capabilities and aptitudes. The impetuous development of the health system requires increasingly better human resources, prepared from the technical, professional and human point of view, who can meet the challenges of scientific-technical development.[13]

The role played by the nursing staff in these services is of vital importance, since their dedication, devotion and high sense of humanism contribute directly to the recovery of patients receiving emergency treatment.

The trust and affection that the population feels for nurses is the result of their dedication, high scientific-technical level and high human sensitivity, which are stimuli achieved by the results of their daily work and the eagerness to improve their individual preparation.

CONCLUSIONS

There are multiple factors that influence the appearance of the threat of preterm labor, a fact that affects the results of the maternal and infant care program. Nursing interventions based on the scientific method will contribute to improve the conditions for delivery, obtaining a newborn with good weight, healthy and without complications.

RECOMMENDATIONS

- ✓ To generalize the proposal for the application of the protocol of care in the threat of preterm labor by nursing personnel, as a working tool in secondary health care, especially in gynecobstetric hospitals.
- ✓ To evaluate the quality of nursing care in patients with threatened preterm labor, once the proposed instrument has been applied.

BIBLIOGRAPHIC REFERENCES

Villar J, Ezcurra EJ, Gurtner de la Fuente V, Campodónico L. Pre-term delivery syndrome: the unmet need. Research & Clinical Forums 2004; 16: 9-33.

2. Keirse MJNC. New perspectives for the effective treatment of preterm labor. Am J Obstet Gynecol 2005;page 173.

3. Rogowski JA. The economics of preterm delivery. Prenat Neonat Med 2008;page 16-20.

4. American College of obstetrician and gynecologist. Management of preterm labor. Washington. DC. American College of obstetrician and gynecologist. 2003.

5. Bettegowda, V.R., et al. The Relationship Between Cesarean Delivery and Gestational Age Among U.S. Singleton Births. Clinics in Perinatology, Volume 35, 2008, pp. 309-323.

6. Health Statistical Yearbook. National Directorate of Medical Records and Health Statistics. 2007.

7. Ministry of Public Health. Infant Mortality Reduction Program. Havana. ECIMED; 2000, p. 36.

8. Savitz D, Blackmore C, Thorp J. Epidemiologic characteristics of preterm delivery etiologic heterogeneity. Am J Obstet Gynecol. 2007; 164: 467-471.

9. National Directorate of Medical Education. Support material for Obstetric Nursing programs. Volume II. Editorial Pueblo y Educación. Havana 1986. 248 - 51.

10. Patient safety. The nurse matters. Press release April 29, 2002 [cited: 12 January 2006]. Available from: http://www.icn.ch/matters_ptsafetysp.htm

11. Nursing in quality control. ACAMI. 2005 [cited: 5 February 2006]. Available from: http://www.acami.org.ar/revista/calidad.htm

12. Ortega C, Suarez M. Nursing quality service evaluation manual. Strategies for its application. Mexico, DF: Editorial Médica Panamericana; 2006.

13. . Benavent MA, et al. Fundamentals of nursing. Spain: DAE. Paradigma Group. Nursing 21; 2000 [cited: 27 January 2006]. Available from: https://www.enfermeria21.com

14. Gilles DA. Nursing management. A systems approach. Barcelona: Mason-Salvat; 2004.

15. . Iyer P. Nursing process and nursing diagnoses. Madrid: Harcourt; 1997.

16. Public Health Statistics Registry. Hospital Materno Norte. 2010.

17. Martin, J.A. et al. Births: Final Data for 2006. National Vital Statistics Reports, volume 57, number 7, January 7, 2008.

18. Calderón G, Vega M. et al. Maternal risk factors associated with preterm birth. Rev. Med. IMSS. 2005, p 43.

19. American College of Obstetricians and Gynecologists (ACOG). Cesarean Delivery on Maternal Request. ACOG Committee Opinion, Number 394, December 2007.

20. Clinical Practice Guidelines. Diagnosis and Management of Partoretérmino. Mexican College of Gynecology and Obstetrics Specialists. 2008. p 129-149.

21. Engle, W.A. and Committee on Fetus and Newborn. Surfactant-Replacement Therapy for Respiratory Distress in the Preterm and Term Neonate. Pediatrics, volume 121, number 2, February 2008, pp. 419-428.

22. Guidelines for the care of patients with threatened preterm labor. 2007. Compañía Suramericana de Servicios de Salud.

23. National Directorate of Medical Education. Support material for Obstetric Nursing programs. Volume II. Editorial Pueblo y Educación. Havana 1986. 248 - 51.

24. Collective of authors. Manual de diagnósticos y tratamiento de Obstetricia y Perinatología. Havana: Editorial Ciencias Médicas; 2005: 1 -365.

25. National Consensus of Perinatology.2010.

26. Althuisius SM, Dekker GA, Hummel, Van Geyn. Cervical incompetence prevention randomized cerclage trial, emergency cerclage with bed res tus bed rest alone. Am I Obstet Gynecol. 2003, page 18.

27. Takai N, Nishida M, Urata K, Yuge A,. Successful cerclage in two patients with advance cervical dilation in the second trimester. Arch Gynecol Obstet. 2003, page 268.

28. Noelia SI. Gynecobstetrician Nursing. Havana. 2009, pg 419

29. Medina Z. Independent nursing actions. Editorial Ciencias Médicas, Havana. 2008. pg 131 - 136.

30. NANDA. NANDA Nursing Diagnoses. Available at: http://www.terra.es/personal/duenas/diagnos.htm.

31. NOC. Nursing diagnosis. https://www.aibarra.org/Apuntes/Fundamentos/Diagnostico%20de%20 Enfermeria.doc

32. Health Books. Nursing Diagnosis. www.librossanitarios.com/detalle.asp?ISBN=844581407-9&codcat=28

33. Limperopoulos, C., et al. Positive Screening for Autism in Ex-Preterm Infants: Prevalence and Risk Factors. Pediatrics, volume 212, number 4, April 2008, pages. 758-765

34. Caballero González J E, Cruz R. Maternal age and its influence on some perinatal disorders. Rev Cubana Obstet y Ginecol.1997; 16(1): 22-8.

35. Puffer RC. Birth weight, maternal age, and birth order. Three important determinants of infant mortality. PAHO. Scientific Publication #298. Washington DC, 2000,94-7.

36. Faundes A. Study of different ways of evaluating maternal weight as indicators of newborn weight. Rev Cubana Obstet Ginecol 2008; 18 (1):25 - 38.

37. Rey, Martinez H. Rational management of the premature infant [Manejo racional del niño prematuro]. I Course of fetal and neonatal medicine. Bogotá, Colombia. 2003:137-51.

38. Reeder Sh I Martin LL, Koniak D. Immediate care of the newborn. In: Enfermería materno infantil 17th edition. Mexico, Editorial Interamericana, SA, 1992. p. 575-594. [online virtual library] http://www.hirv.Mc.master.ca/org

39. Legault M, Goulet C. Comparison of kangaroo and traditional methods of removing preterm infants from incubators. J Obstet Gynecol Neonatal Nurs 2005; 24: 501-6.

40. Honein, M.A., et al. The Association Between Major Birth Defects and Preterm Birth. Maternal and Child Health Journal, published online May 17, 2008. https://:dx/doi/org/10.1007.s10995-0080348-y.

Alvarez Fumero A. Impact of risk factors on low birth weight. Rev Summary 2001; 14 (13):115-21.

ANNEXES

Annex No. 1 Patient informed consent.

I: ______________________________ have met and agree to participate in the research related to procedures that the nurse will perform on me to improve my health, it will not cause me physical or social harm or prejudice and I may leave the study at any time.

Signature: _______________

Annex No. 2 Data collection form.

No. __________ Medical History _________

1. Date of entry _________

2. Age.

   ✓ Under 18 years old_________
   ✓ 19-35 years_________
   ✓ Over 35 years old _________

3. Parity

   ✓ Primipara________
   ✓ Multipara________

4. Mother's occupation

   ✓ Homemaker_________
   ✓ Worker_________
   ✓ Student_________

5. Marital status

   ✓ Single_________
   ✓ Married_________

6. Gestational age

   ✓ Between 27 and 34 weeks_________
   ✓ Between 34.1 and 36.6 weeks_________

7. Weight of the newborn

   ✓ Less than 2500 grams_________
   ✓ Greater than 2500 grams________

8. Diseases associated with pregnancy

- ✓ Anemias ________
- ✓ Cervical vaginal infections________
- ✓ Urinary tract infections________
- ✓ Hypertensive disease________
- ✓ Cervical incompetence________
- ✓ Retroplacental hematoma________
- ✓ Coriamnionitis________
- ✓ Premature rupture of membranes________

9. Obstetric history

- ✓ Early primiparity________
- ✓ Previous spontaneous preterm labor________
- ✓ Previous induced abortions________
- ✓ Previous miscarriages in the second half of the year ________
- ✓ Twin pregnancy________
- ✓ Low size________
- ✓ Poor socioeconomic conditions________
- ✓ Toxic habits________
- ✓ Short intergenesis periods________
- ✓ Others________

10. Did you have any adverse reaction to the medication applied?

- ✓ Yes________
- ✓ No ________
- ✓ Cuál

____

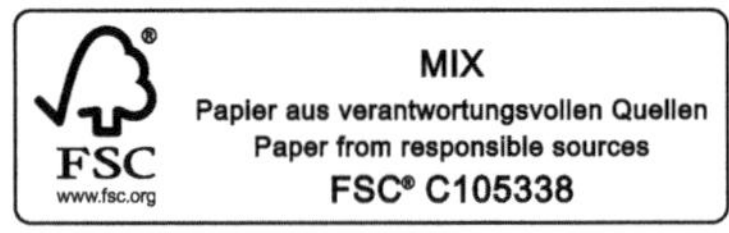

Printed by Books on Demand GmbH, Norderstedt / Germany